ANGER-GRIEF
the JESUS Way

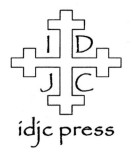

idjc press

Anger-Grief the Jesus Way
Copyright 2009
Stephen Joseph Wolf

Contact idjc press at steve@idjc.info.

Cover art by the author

Printed in the U.S.A.

ISBN 978-0-9795549-2-6

Anger-Grief the Jesus Way
is available at ST. MARY'S BOOKSTORE
1919 West End Avenue, Nashville, TN 37203
www.stmarysbookstore.com

Dedicated to Father Ryan High School's
Humbert Aloysius "Pat" Corsini
who suffered my slow progress in the French language
while teaching me to love the good story

AS ABBA LOVES

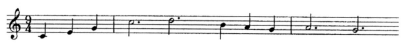

1. As Ab - ba loves me   so do I love you.
2. I am the vine and   you are my bran - ches;
3. No great - er love than   has one to lay down
4. You have been with me   from the be - gin - ing;

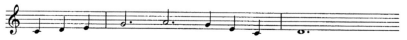

1. I tell you this: re - main in my   love.
2. Let Ab -ba prune you so you bear   fruit.
3. One's ve - ry life for e - ven a   friend.
4. Tes - ti - fy in the Spi - rit of   truth.

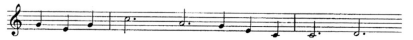

1. Keep this co - mand - ment:
2. My word re - mem - ber:
3. You I have cho - sen: Love one an - oth - er
4. In word and ac - tion:

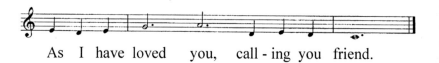

As I have loved you, call - ing you friend.

A tribute to the priesthood of Rev.Charley Giacosa

Text:from John 15, Stephen J. Wolf, 2007

Music: BUNESSAN 5554 D, Scots Gaelic melody, Popular: *Morning Has Broken*

Previously published in *Psalm Songs.*

Used with permission.

ANGER-GRIEF the JESUS Way

INTRODUCTION: The Story

Sabbath is the day of the week. Jesus is in the synagogue in Capernaum. Others are there, including some Pharisees and a silent man with a withered hand. Jesus knows the Pharisees are wondering if he will break the law again by healing on the Sabbath. He asks them a riddle, to engage them in dialogue. They remain silent, refusing to talk to him. He turns to them in anger and is grieved at their hardness of heart. He then asks the silent man to stretch out his withered hand, and it is healed. The Pharisees go out to make plans how best to kill him.

The story itself is one of those readings in our three-year Sunday Lectionary cycle often omitted, knocked out by an early Lent. So it is a story we hear on Sundays less than once every three years. And it is not chosen for special feast days.

The Son of God experienced human anger. He was aware of the unhealed or willful block in the Pharisees that kept them from entering into dialogue with him. God invites and cajoles, but God does not violate our freedom. So in his humanity, Jesus feels

---

* Mark 3:1-6, on the Ninth Sunday of Year B, Ordinary Time.

the emotion of anger. In his divinity he loves even
these Pharisees. He wants to engage them in some
kind of healing dialogue, but they refuse in stubborn
silence. He acknowledges to himself this human
emotion of anger, and then holds it with grief, with
divine compassion. He suffers with the Pharisees who
are still unhealed, still blocked.

In Chapter 3, Verse 5, of the Gospel of Mark, we
have the only passage in the New Testament in which
we are told that Jesus experienced the emotion of
anger.

About what might this be? I have been told that
depression is anger turned inward. I know something
about depression, the way you know something about
your cross. You know, the one you have been called
by Jesus to pick up daily and carry while following him.

I suppose my depression cross is why they invited
me in the seminary to take a look at my "anger issue."
I had to admit it. I have an anger issue. I have my
sainted mother's Scotch-Irish temper. But I was a holy
seminarian! How could they tell I had an anger issue?

No matter. Filled with the glow of a new Bible
student with matter for exegesis, I headed straight for

the concordance. *Exegesis. Concordance.* Two new words in my vocabulary. The concordance would give me a list of every time the word *anger* (or *angry*) is used in the Bible. I wanted to know something about Jesus and anger. Only one passage applied:

Mark 3:5   *...looking around at them with* **anger** *...*

Surely, this was not the only passage that used the word anger or angry and applied it to Jesus! What about, you might be thinking as I was, what about Jesus cleansing the temple? He drove them out with a whip! I know he was angry that day!

So I read all four accounts of the temple cleansing scene: Mark 11:15-19; Matthew 21:12-13; Luke 19:45-46; John 2:14-16. John's version skirts closest to anger, but we're told he went to the trouble of making a whip. When I slow down to be a craftsman, my anger usually slides away in the work. But John does mention the whip, a weapon:

...Jesus went up to Jerusalem. He found in the temple area those who sold oxen, sheep, and doves, as well as the money-changers seated there. He made a whip out of cords and drove them all

out of the temple area, with the sheep and oxen,
and spilled the coins of the money-changers and
overturned their tables, and to those who sold doves
he said, "Take these out of here,
and stop making my Father's house a marketplace."
His disciples recalled the words of scripture,
"Zeal for your house will consume me."

John 2:13b-17 (*Zeal* is from Psalm 69:10)

Zeal. Not the same thing as anger. Experiment
with this passage in your imagination. In John, this is
right after the first sign at the Cana wedding. Pretend
that Jesus knows fully well that it is time to draw some
attention to himself and begin challenging the status
quo. Imagine that Jesus knows that in the progression
of his ministry those with power and authority would
have to get riled up at him. Knowing that some anger
among them was inevitable, what if Jesus had the
most enjoyable day of his three years of teaching and
preaching and healing? Have you ever pushed your
best friends' buttons, just to rile them up, just for fun,
or even for their own good?

When my seven brothers and I were young boys,
and one of us would ask our father, "Hey Deddy, *

* We spelled "Deddy" the same way we said it.

5

why are you doing this?" His favorite non-answer was "funzies," just for fun. Praying once with one of these temple passages, I watched Jesus fashion a whip to use, looking at me with a face expressive of "watch this!" I had already read the passage, so I knew the purpose of the whip. When I asked Jesus why, he answered, "funzies." Like a parent trying to discipline a child, or a friend at play with a practical joke, Jesus could not let them see him laughing inside. So the effect on the crowd was the same. Inside jokes can be the best, and zeal can be funny too.

Well, what about when Jesus rebuked Simon, even calling him Satan! Surely Simon made him mad! In Mark, this happens after the first of three predictions of Jesus' coming passion and death.* We are told simply that Simon *rebuked* Jesus and that Jesus then *rebuked* Simon, looking at his disciples saying "Get behind me, Satan. You are thinking not as God does, but as human beings do." In Matthew, Jesus also calls Peter *an obstacle* to him. Luke lets his friend Peter off the hook, levelling the *rebuke* by Jesus against all the apostles, directing them to tell no one who Jesus is.

* Mark 8:31-33; see also Matthew 16:21-27; Luke 9:22-26.

Again, as in the cleansing of the temple, Jesus may indeed have been angry with Peter, but the gospel writers do not use that word. The setting and the tone suggest *anger,* but the word is not used.

And this is my point in this introduction:

The gospel narrative does tell us, with the word, that Jesus was angry, but only once, and by only one gospel writer (Mark), and in only one episode (3:1-6, the story of the healing of the man with a withered hand). It is certainly reasonable to suggest that, in events similar to the cleansing of the temple and Jesus' rebuke of Peter, our Lord was angry, and that those around him knew he was angry. All four authors, including Mark, did not choose to use the word.

Why are we told of it in this particular passage? Why in this specific story? Might the Holy Spirit be trying to tell us something in this explicit account of the human anger of Jesus the Christ? I think so, and I think I know what.

1   *Again Jesus entered the synagogue.*
There was a man there
who had a withered hand.

2   *They watched him closely*
to see if he would cure him on the sabbath
so that they might accuse him.

3   *He said to the man with the withered hand,*
"Come up here before us."

4   *Then he said to them,*
"Is it lawful to do good on the sabbath
rather than to do evil,
to save life rather than destroy it?"
But they remained silent.

5   *Looking around at them with anger*
and grieved at their hardness of heart,
he said to the man,
"Stretch out your hand."
He stretched it out and his hand was restored.

6   *The Pharisees went out*
and immediately took counsel with the Herodians
against him to put him to death.

Mark 3:1-6

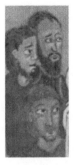

I

A Sabbath Assembly

Again Jesus entered the synagogue.
There was a man there
who had a withered hand.   Mark 3:1

Again. Jesus had crossed this threshhold for what,
30 years? How many sabbaths is that? There was a
day when he could do so as one of the crowd, hardly
being noticed. Not any more, unless he is able to go
into a church, synagogue or mosque in this third
millenium without being noticed. Do Christians hold
him to his promise of Matthew 18:20?

For where two or three (or more?) *are gathered*
in my name, there am I in the midst of them.

9

If two is company and three is a crowd, then two is also private, and three (or more) is public. When we gather in the name of Jesus, whether in private or in public, there he is, in our midst, a real presence. Is this why our liturgy calls for an Opening Song, to proclaim out loud *both* that we are gathered in his name *and* that God is with us, Emmanuel?

We are told that he was in the habit of entering the synagogue. I've heard it said that forming a new habit takes 40 times, or 28 days, or 6 weeks, before the thing is no longer new, but ingrained. Entering the assembly is what Jesus did, and what Jesus does.

We know that the synagogue service was not the same as the temple sacrifices, synagogues having been built wherever there was a community of faithful Jews, and there being only one true temple, the one in Jerusalem. Since early in the first millenium, there have been four parts to the Christian Sunday liturgy: ① gather in, ② proclaim the word, ③ break the bread, and ④ go forth on mission. Liturgists have compared the synagogue service of Jesus' day with our Liturgy of the Word, and the temple sacrifice of Jesus' day with our Liturgy of the Eucharist.

Our very word "Church" is a translation of the Greek word *ekklesia* (Mt 16:18;18:17), for the Hebrew word for the assembly of the chosen people in the 40 years of desert pilgrimage from Egypt to the Promised Land, after being led out of slavery and before being led into freedom. Our church still wanders, but as pilgrims, not nomads. As with the chosen people in the exodus, God has for us a destination.

An important distinction is that our Sunday is not the Sabbath day of rest marked by our Jesus, the faithful Jew, or for his disciples and apostles in the earliest days of the church. Since the Sabbath, the seventh day of the week, was the day of rest for the people of Jerusalem, the experience of the earliest churches might have been similar to us taking the day of rest on Sunday, and then going to weekly Mass before going to work on Monday. I am told that just a couple of generations before me, many Catholic Irish in Nashville had to work on Sundays, and so would attend the dawn mass at Cathedral of the Incarnation, and then go to work. Is their experience all that different from that of early Christians or third millenium immigrants?

It is important for Christians to remember that we do what we do on Sundays *on Sunday* because Sunday is the day on which Easter happened, the first day of the week. Every Sunday is another Easter, and it is the resurrection that makes all the difference.

But back to Jesus of Nazareth, now of Capernaum, who enters the synagogue with everyone's eyes upon him. Their eyes are also on another: a man there who has a withered hand.

There are two problems: (1) The man has a real disability, just like others who have already been healed by Jesus. (2) The decalogue: *Remember to keep holy the sabbath day* (Exodus 20:8), the day of rest.

Is it the man's right hand or left hand? We are not told. We can presume that it is a problem for him, for if the withered hand was not experienced by the man as a problem, why would he need a cure?

The problem may be as simple as the competition of the day-laborer. We are told in the previous passage that the fields of grain are ready with heads of grain. With only one good hand, he would be one of the last workers to be hired. He would only be hired if there was a shortage of workers, and he would not be able to harvest as much grain as other workers. When times are difficult and a day-laborer is not hired, it may come down to no work means no pay, means no food to eat, or the indignity of being a charity case.

We are not told whether the withering has been for his whole life or only recently. It really does not matter. Jesus has already been healing many people.

A SABBATH ASSEMBLY

Clearly this man's withered hand is suitable matter for the ministry of Jesus.

We are also not told that the man asks to be healed, or that he has a friend or family member who makes the request. Perhaps this is an indication of the isolation that his malady has brought upon him.

So what about the hand? I have an early memory of doing simple yard work with Momma and some of my brothers. It was at the old house, so I was no older than ten. I wanted the hoe being used by a brother, and said so. Momma paused in her work, and after a quick look told me to just use my hands. My hands? She told me to look at my hands and said, "Nobody has invented any tool better than those two that God has already given you." My hands became a treasure.

A man in the parish is missing one of his thumbs. He once told me that people have no idea what a gift it is to have "opposable digits."

What kinds of stories might this synagogue man be able to tell of how one hand, be it withered or be it healed, can make a huge difference?

If I forget you, Jerusalem, may my right hand wither.
Psalm 137:5

1   *Again Jesus entered the synagogue.*
     There was a man there who had a withered hand.
2   **They watched him closely**
     to see if he would cure him on the sabbath
     so that they might accuse him.
3   *He said to the man with the withered hand,*
     "Come up here before us."
4   *Then he said to them,*
     "Is it lawful to do good on the sabbath
     rather than to do evil,
     to save life rather than destroy it?"
     But they remained silent.
5   *Looking around at them with anger*
     and grieved at their hardness of heart,
     he said to the man,
     "Stretch out your hand."
     He stretched it out and his hand was restored.
6   *The Pharisees went out*
     and immediately took counsel with the Herodians
     against him to put him to death.

                                    Mark 3:1-6

14

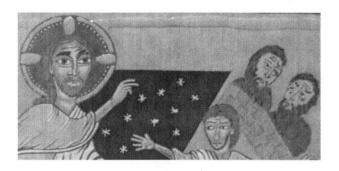

II

Being Watched

They watched him closely
to see if he would cure him on the sabbath
so that they might accuse him.

Mark 3:2

I have a friend who once told someone "In me, you have an enemy to the grave!" My friend died. At the funeral visitation, another friend wanted to remind the man to whom those words had been spoken that, "he's not in the grave yet!"

Do you know someone who might presume to consider himself or herself to be your enemy? Is there someone you sometimes consider to be your enemy?

If I directed this question about you to your spouse, boss, doctor, lawyer, mother, son, business partner, golf buddy, bunko sister, massage therapist, dentist, barber, hairdresser, brother monk, sister nun, closest neighbor or best friend, would one of them be able to help you name that person? (I sometimes ask the child who can't think in the confessional of even one sin, "is there something your mother might want you remember?") I do ask you to reflect on a time in your life when you experienced having an enemy. How did that come about?

There is always a background story. Here is the background for our Anger-Grief story:

Back again to Jesus, who enters the synagogue with everyone's eyes on him. We are still early in the concise account of *the gospel of Jesus Christ the Son of God* (Mark 1:1). Already Jesus has been baptized in the Jordan by John, hearing the voice from the heavens: *You are my beloved Son; with you I am well pleased;* been driven by the Spirit into the desert for forty days and been tempted; begun to proclaim in Galilee *the gospel of God:*

> *This is the time of fulfillment.*
> *The kingdom of God is at hand.*
> *Repent, and believe in the gospel.*   Mark 1:15

He has called the two sets of brother-fishermen: Simon and Andrew, James and John; in Capernaum on a sabbath he cured a man with an unclean spirit and Simon's mother-in-law, and after the sabbath-ending sunset cured *many who were sick with various diseases* (1:34), and he drove out many demons.

After a very early morning of prayer, he left Capernaum, but cleansed a begging leper, who then *began to publicize the whole matter...so that it was impossible for Jesus to enter a town openly.* He stayed in deserted places, but *people kept coming to him from everywhere* (1:45).

After some days, Jesus went back to Capernaum and we have a sort of shift in the tone, where Jesus becomes more provocative.

Word spread, a crowd gathered, and he *preached the word to them* (2:2). Into the middle of this a paralytic is carried by four men, whose faith inspires Jesus to say to the paralytic,

Child, your sins are forgiven (2:5).

Now he has the attention of *some of the scribes* there, who begin asking each other if Jesus is blaspheming. We are told that Jesus knows *in his mind what they were thinking to themselves* (2:8). He asks them a rhetorical question, and without waiting for a response declares

> *"that you may know that the Son of Man*
> *has authority to forgive sins on earth"*
> *he said to the paralytic,*
> *"I say to you, rise, pick up your mat, and go home."*

The paralytic does as Jesus said, and all are
astounded.

The crowd follows him along the sea, and he
teaches them. He calls Levi, who leaves his customs
job and feeds Jesus in his own house. Some *scribes*
who were Pharisees see Jesus eating with *sinners and tax*
collectors, and challenge not Jesus but his disciples.
Jesus himself hears their questioning and responds,

> *"Those who are well do not need a physician,*
> *but the sick do. I did not come to call the righteous*
> *but sinners. (2:17).*

When people question Jesus about his disciples not
fasting as did the disciples of John and the Pharisees,
Jesus answers with parables of wedding guests with
the bridegroom and new wine in new wineskins.
When Jesus teaches in parables, we know there are

always multiple layers of meaning.

The Pharisees themselves then challenge Jesus directly with the bad example given by his hungry disciples, who pick heads of grain ("work") on a sabbath while walking through a field. He responds with the unimpeachable example of King David himself and his companions, who violated the law by eating the bread of offering in the house of God, and then gives them this blunt mystery:

> "*The sabbath was made for man,*
> *not man for the sabbath.*
> *That is why the Son of Man*
> *is lord even of the sabbath.*" Mark 2:27b,28

This language is very dangerous to a whole way of life built not just on the Torah, but around all kinds of other rules of life. If the weekly observance of the sabbath was up for grabs, what would be next? If the *scribes who are Pharisees* have a response to what Jesus has just said, we are not told it.

So, here we are again in the synagogue on another sabbath. Jesus enters again.

1 *Again Jesus entered the synagogue.*
There was a man there who had a withered hand.

2 *They watched him closely*
to see if he would cure him on the sabbath
so that they might accuse him.

3 **He said to the man with the withered hand,**
"Come up here before us."

4 *Then he said to them,*
"Is it lawful to do good on the sabbath
rather than to do evil,
to save life rather than destroy it?"
But they remained silent.

5 *Looking around at them with anger*
and grieved at their hardness of heart,
he said to the man,
"Stretch out your hand."
He stretched it out and his hand was restored.

6 *The Pharisees went out*
and immediately took counsel with the Herodians
against him to put him to death.

Mark 3:1-6

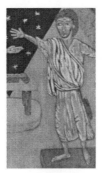

III

Invited By Jesus

He said to the man with the withered hand,
"Come up here before us."

Mark 3:3

St. Ignatius of Loyola suggests a way to pray with
scripture, especially around gospel stories with action.
This way, from his *Spiritual Exercises,* is to let the gospel
account be as an outline, presuming that the gospel
writers never tell us everything that happened. For
example, was it sunny, cloudy or rainy? Hot, cold,
dry, humid? Are there noises or silence? Is there any
music or background noise or conversation? What is
on the minds of the people in the story? Can we tell

21

whether it is indoors or outdoors? What kind of mood
are Jesus and the disciples in? Is there anything there
to eat or drink? Is anyone hungry or thirsty?

OK, sometimes we are told some of these things,
but never everything. St. Ignatius suggests that we
familiarize ourselves enough with the outline provided
in the gospel account, taking seriously what is there,
and then place our very self into the story, as one of
the actual characters.

When I pray this way, I usually try to be just a
bystander, part of the crowd. But Jesus almost always
makes me play the part of Peter or whoever the other
main character is. When praying this particular story,
the Lord has so far let me rest in the nervous antici-
pation of the synagogue crowd.

Try St. Ignatius' *exercise* sometime when you have
thirty minutes or an hour. Give yourself over to the
story, and let your imagination pray through all your
senses: sight, sound, smell, touch, hearing, and even
your intuition. But just let the whole story unfold.
Let the Father and the Son through the Holy Spirit
speak through the sacred word to your inmost being.

Have you ever been invited to a party to which
you did not want to go? Have you ever been called
to stand in front of a public gathering without any

warning? Put yourself in the place of the man.

I have sometimes prayed this passage where the man with the withered hand is new to the community and does not know anything about Jesus. He is very uncertain of responding to his call to front and center.

Another time, the man has been away during all of the early activity, and though he has heard about this healer, this is the first time he has seen him. He is hopeful that he can heal him, and would ask him if given the opportunity. Another time the hand had been withered since birth. Still another time, the withering was from a recent accident.

This hasn't happened, but I wonder if it ever will: In the wonderfully irreverent Monty Python movie *Life of Brian,* a beggar is bouncing around Brian, asking for alms for the poor. Brian tells the beggar that there is nothing to keep him from working, so stop bothering people and go get a job.

The man said, "I used to have a job. I was a crippled beggar. And then this Jesus came by and cured me. Took away my livelihood, he did."
The exasperated Brian finally gives the bouncing beggar a coin to get rid of him, and in mock gratitude, the beggar said, "Oh, half a shekel! Thank you very much!" to which Brian replied, "there's no pleasing

some people." The beggar bounces off out loud,
"that's the same thing that Jesus said!"

Some of us with something withered do not want
to be healed. We have grown used to our infirmity,
thank you very much, and do not want any kind of
change.

There is a difference between seeking a cure and
learning to cope. I cannot be cured of the fact that I
will someday die, so I learn to cope with it. If dying
is our universal fear, it is the root of all other fears.
We humans have tried all kinds of coping mechanisms:
deny; make the best of things; *eat and drink and enjoy
the fruit of all (our) labor* (Ecclesiastes 3:13); ancestor
worship; try to live forever by amassing enough power,
wealth, or the perfect diet or exercise to build what
Lutheran Ted Peters calls a *citadel of psychic safety* or
live in what Paul Tillich called *self-complacent finitude*
(two country music songs just begging to be written).
And there will always be people around, themselves
in denial, to help us stay distracted in methods that
offer no cure but plenty of pretense and coping.

As a Christian, I want to argue that on Easter
Sunday, Christ did overcome death and so we have
the cure to all our fear. Alas, we are still human. As
a parishioner once put it so well, "I'm not afraid of

death; I'm afraid of *the dying,* you know, the pain."
When I quote Daffy Duck, "I don't like pain; it hurts
me; I'm not like other people," I am most certainly
using humor as my favorite coping mechanism.

So, the man with the withered hand was invited
to stand front and center, to bring his most urgent
need for healing to Jesus. *So what (!)* if Jesus wants to
to make a point even broader than that he can heal.
So what (!) if the man is being used by Jesus as a visual
aid to teach something to these scribes. *So what (!)* if
the work that Jesus wants to accomplish in me is
never only about or for me alone.

Once while praying this story, I was on the edge
of the crowd, into which Jesus disappeared. He
popped up behind me and pulled me into the field of
grain to laugh in private about how the Pharisees had
acted, but was also sad that they could not give themselves permission to see the good things that God
wanted to do in their lives. Still, he loved them.

Someday, I don't know when, I expect to pray
this passage as the man with the withered hand.
When I do, I expect to find out what it is that Christ
wants to heal in me, the thing I don't even know is
withered. Funny thing, I can ask for this grace now!
I wonder why I don't.

1   *Again Jesus entered the synagogue.*
    There was a man there who had a withered hand.
2   *They watched him closely*
    to see if he would cure him on the sabbath
    so that they might accuse him.
3   *He said to the man with the withered hand,*
    "Come up here before us."
4   ***Then he said to them,***
    "Is it lawful to do good on the sabbath
    rather than to do evil,
    to save life rather than destroy it?"
    But they remained silent.
5   *Looking around at them with anger*
    and grieved at their hardness of heart,
    he said to the man,
    "Stretch out your hand."
    He stretched it out and his hand was restored.
6   *The Pharisees went out*
    and immediately took counsel with the Herodians
    against him to put him to death.

                                        Mark 3:1-6

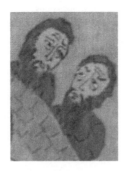

IV

Riddle Silence

Then he said to them,
"Is it lawful to do good on the sabbath
rather than to do evil,
to save life rather than destroy it?"
But they remained silent.

Mark 3:4

I don't like to play games. I suppose it is because games with my seven brothers almost always broke out in fights. One by one, every board game, electric football, mechanical basketball, every toy that involved a game disappeared mysteriously. I can't ask her now until heaven, but I'm pretty sure Momma absconded them all, like an efficient warden. There is a distant memory of her so much as admitting to one instance. Of course, this was for our own good, to help us live in peace. We invented our own. *Balloonsketball,* for example, was played with a balloon and a wire clothes hanger, bent into a hoop and hung over a door. It was a game you could play in silence when grounded.

So, I don't like to play games. And I don't like riddles.

Jesus, my Lord and Savior, likes riddles. And so, I sometimes pray with his riddles.

They, the Pharisees who are also in the synagogue, well, it seems that they do not like riddles either. My suspicion is that their teachers in pharisee school used riddles as part of their technique, and that they enjoyed it as much as I enjoyed teachers who used the so-called socratic method of debate teaching, which was not at all. Introverts consider it torture.

And so, they remained silent. They gave Jesus the stone face. I know how to do that. I give it to the parishioner who is lambasting me about something, or the visitor who wishes to tell me in subtext that he or she is more holy than anyone in our parish, or the speaker who talks out of assumptions he or she thinks no one would dare to challenge as unorthodox. The stone face is a coping mechanism that helps me to keep an inner explosion from tipping into a tantrum of temper. The stone face is also a defensive power ploy, an attempt to say to the source of the inner boiling that, "you know, you really do not have this power you think you have over me." The stone face does not always work. Sometimes temper wins.

I suspect that the Pharisees were using the tactic of the stone face. Is there any other reason for their silence?

History might have something to tell us in the *Letter of the Pharisee,* recently discovered in a box of old seminary homework:

Brothers and sisters in Christ, when you asked me some weeks ago about my life as a Pharisee, I thought it best to reflect on how best to explain my former identity. The Greek word 'pharisaioi' seems to be based on the Aramaic 'perisaye' and the Hebrew 'perusim,' which means the 'separated ones.' We are not sure about its source, but it likely came from some of our detractors. We accepted being labelled as 'the separate ones' because we saw it as our role to be an example, to be separated from those who are not yet following the law, the Torah. You see, we were good Jews, devout and pious. We were not ordained or anointed, but were recognized by our piety and by our serious study. Our roots may have been in the 'scribes' of the law. We were educated and emphasized knowledge and a strict interpretation of the Torah. This separated us, making us different from most of our kinsfolk who could not read or write. But we were not separated in our common goal: to be a holy nation, sacred and dedicated to Yahweh. Also, while the priests served God in the Jerusalem Temple, we were called to serve in our way of life. Our prayer was not limited to the temple sacrifice. But we were very aware of what the priests did there. We watched the sacrifices to help make sure that ritual purity was maintained. Though all of the law given in the Torah was indispensible, we came to be marked as very strictly observing the sabbath, ritual purity regulations, and tithing. We made no apologies about this. We were proud of these observances as part of our Judean ancestry. We often had great influence in political and social matters, though some of our number may have involved themselves too much in secular matters. Most of our focus was pointing out violations of the law. We were accused by some of writing our own laws, of doing what should only be done by the Lord. It was true that we relied on oral tradition as well as the written Torah, but that was to help people avoid breaching the Torah. Let me explain. In the normal course of life, a faithful Jew may set out to obey the Torah, living each moment completely aware of its precepts. By our count there are 613 separate laws in the Torah. The laws might not be clear to a devoted but unsophisticated Jew, who would therefore benefit from a system of rituals of life. Our rituals were meant to include the Torah plus other helpful ways to obey the Torah. They could be seen as a kind of fence around the law. The fence helped give people assurance of being faithful to the Torah itself. We felt we were serving the people by giving example and guidance in a way of life accessible to all, resulting in obedience to the Torah. There can be no question that the Sabbath was observed more faithfully due to our influence. We also dealt with the critical question of the Messiah; we waited with all of Judea. We Pharisees considered it our duty to look for him with vigilance. The prophets told us he would be a descendent of David (Isaiah 11:2-5). We expected he would be the royal savior, the one who would restore Israel to power. Until the Messiah came, we accepted it as the will of Yahweh that we remain under Roman rule. Our role was to help find the Messiah and to make him known to the people. We also rooted out false messiahs, and there were many of them. We were confident that when the Messiah came, we would recognize him. As you know, in this we failed.

1   *Again Jesus entered the synagogue.*
      There was a man there who had a withered hand.

2   *They watched him closely*
      to see if he would cure him on the sabbath
      so that they might accuse him.

3   *He said to the man with the withered hand,*
      "Come up here before us."

4   *Then he said to them,*
      "Is it lawful to do good on the sabbath
      rather than to do evil,
      to save life rather than destroy it?"
      But they remained silent.

5   ***Looking around at them with anger***
      and grieved at their hardness of heart,
      he said to the man,
      "Stretch out your hand."
      He stretched it out and his hand was restored.

6   *The Pharisees went out*
      and immediately took counsel with the Herodians
      against him to put him to death.

                             Mark 3:1-6

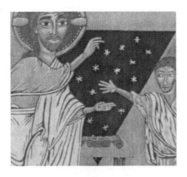

V

Anger-Grief

Looking around at them with anger
and grieved at their hardness of heart,
he said to the man,
"Stretch out your hand."
He stretched it out
and his hand was restored.

Mark 3:5

So, here's the word. *Anger.* The gospel of Mark tells us that Jesus was angry.

If you have hung in this long, you may have gone to your dictionary by now. Let's take a look.

33

These are from an old *Webster's New World Dict-ionary* in a Trappist monastery guest house library:

an.ger (ang'ger), *n.* a feeling of being very annoyed and wanting to fight back at a person or thing that hurts one or is against one; wrath; rage.

grief (gref), *n.* 1. deep and painful sorrow, as that caused by someone's death. 2. something that causes such sorrow. -**come to grief**, to fail or be ruined.

Anger is an emotion. Say it out loud: *Anger is an emotion.* It is not imaginary; it is real. It is like hunger and thirst: anger is part of our animal nature. Like hunger and thirst, anger is a feeling that first comes *to* us, arrives at the scene, almost always as a surprise visitor. Free will enters when we choose what we *do* with it. But before we can *choose* what to do with it, we have to become *aware* that the emotion of anger is upon us. Am I able to recognize an arrival of anger?

I think that Jesus is showing us through this story how this process of *awareness* then *choice* can unfold.

Like you and me, Jesus is a human being, fully human. Fully human and fully divine. Fully God and fully man. As a teacher Eugene LaVerdiere liked to put it, "not God on his Poppa's side and human on his Momma's side," understood by some incorrectly as half God and half man. No, we proclaim Jesus as fully God and fully human. OK, the Church argued quite a bit and quite vehemently before we came to a concensus about how best to speak of the two natures of Christ. The result uses 20 of the 32 lines that make up the Nicene Creed, formulated for the most part at the Council of Nicea in 325 A.D.

The Greek word used in Mark 3:5, οργη, could probably be translated as *wrath* instead of *anger*. We tend to think of *wrath* as a word to use for the divine, as in *the wrath of God*. If the gospel writer is pointing to the humanity of Jesus, we can see it in the use of the word *anger,* and in the very telling itself of this story of Jesus failing.

Remember, the gospel of Mark was written in perhaps around 75 A.D. for a community undergoing persecution, and so dealing with their own difficulties. Mark has been called *a passion narrative with a prologue.* An unexpected failure can be a powerful prompter of the anger emotion. Perhaps Jesus is angry about his own inability to break through to the pharisees, to win them over so they can see his side of the story.

Every preacher wants converts. Few experiences give me as much simple selfish joy as when a fellow Christian who still agrees with using the death penalty steps up after mass to report, even as one retired police officer recently put it with his forefinger and thumb almost touching in the air between us, "Father, you *almost* had me that time." This was big.

My suspicion is that the source of the emotion of anger in our story is the silence of the pharisees. They will not even talk to him. They will talk *about* him, but they refuse to enter into dialogue with Jesus. And this makes him hopping mad.

There are two reasons that I suggest Mark 3:1-6 as a penance in the sacrament of reconciliation when a person expresses the desire to be healed of anger. The first reason is the gospel truth that in his humanity Jesus too was angry. The second reason is what he does in this story with his anger. He grieves.

His grief is over their hardness of heart. The root of the Greek word for *hardness* is πωροω, or *poroo,* pronounced *po-ro'-o,* apparently from πωρος or *poros* (a kind of stone); to *petrify,* that is, (figuratively) to *indurate (render stupid* or *callous):* -blind, harden.

Their hearts, made by God to be beating, living, had become in them petrified, like stone, by their own

choice, it seems. They have already been losing these
battles of wits with Jesus, so it is easier to give a stubborn stone face that reflects the hard heart. They
won't lose if they refuse to play the game.

We are not told what it is that Jesus sees in their
heart. We were told four episodes earlier, in the
event with the paralytic, that Jesus *knew in his mind
what they were thinking to themselves.* How frightened
must they have become when they heard Jesus say out
loud, *why are you thinking such things in your hearts?* (2:8).
Perhaps this is why they remained silent when faced
with his riddle, scared to tangle with one who knows
their own thoughts and feelings. Is that a fair fight?

Here we are faced with the difference between
Jesus and me. OK, there are **many** ways that I am
unlike Jesus; OK, admitted. So here is one difference
between Jesus and me: I can never really know what
is going on in the heart of another human being. How
sadly unaware am I of how my own heart moves! This
is why to judge is the job of God alone, who searches
the mind and knows the heart (Psalms 7:10b, 94:11,
and all of Psalm 139). We humans lack the insight to
judge each other well. Jesus can look into the human
heart and see desires, motivations, imperfections,
and blockages. Like an X-ray that can see a blocked

artery, Jesus can see a stone wall erected in a heart.
So why doesn't he just break down that wall, explode
that stumbling block? An answer is in God's respect
for our freedom. Freedom means that we can choose
to love God, and that we can choose to not love God.
Freedom matters; we are not robots. When we love
God, it matters that we do so freely and not as slaves.

Here we have a big-time paradox. The saints
define freedom as the capacity to say only *yes* to God.
When I say this to young adults, they give me the
turned-head look that a young dog gives when you
make a funny noise, or they stare defiantly at the man
they now consider a communist standing there (me).
I am not a communist. And I don't play one on TV.

The saints are getting at this: As long as I am
unable to say *yes* to God, then I am still somehow
enslaved to something other than God. I am not yet
free. Saintly freedom, then, is not the blessing of
many options, but the grace to know which of them
is the one God desires that I choose. As the Trappist
monk Thomas Merton put it, when I am in touch with
God's deepest desire for me then I am in touch with
my deepest and most real desire for myself. To be
able to choose accordingly is to be free.

These pharisees are not free. The stone wall in

their hearts reflected in the stone wall on their faces
might have been built by them of their own free will.
Who in that synagogue could know the desires,
motivations, imperfections and blockages of those
pharisees? God alone. Jesus, in his divinity, sees
all of it, even the blockages to which they are blind.
He wants to heal them. But God will not violate
our freedom. In his divinity, Jesus will not force his
healing on them, and in his humanity he fails to cajole
them into freedom. For some reason, they will not
enter into dialogue with him. Anger rises within our
Lord, and he turns to them.

What does he then do with his anger? He is
grieved. He holds the emotion of anger with grief.
He holds the humanity of his anger in his divine hand
of compassion. He does the same thing that is so
often the only thing God can do with us: compassion.
He *suffers with.*

And that man with the withered hand? Jesus asks
him to do what the pharisees were unwilling or unfree
to do, to **stretch** . The man does stretch out his hand,
a gesture like Mary's *fiat,* her *yes,* and he is made
whole, restored to the way he was created in God's
image. He can throw away his coping skills, because
he is cured.

1   *Again Jesus entered the synagogue.*
There was a man there who had a withered hand.

2   *They watched him closely*
to see if he would cure him on the sabbath
so that they might accuse him.

3   *He said to the man with the withered hand,*
"Come up here before us."

4   *Then he said to them,*
"Is it lawful to do good on the sabbath
rather than to do evil,
to save life rather than destroy it?"
But they remained silent.

5   *Looking around at them with anger*
and grieved at their hardness of heart,
he said to the man,
"Stretch out your hand."
He stretched it out and his hand was restored.

6   **The Pharisees went out**
and immediately took counsel
with the Herodians against him
to put him to death.

Mark 3:1-6

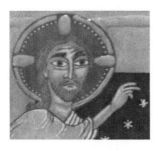

VI

Turning To Freedom

*The Pharisees went out
and immediately took counsel
with the Herodians against him
to put him to death.*

Mark 3:6

We are told how this little story ends. These pharisees, toward whom Jesus feels both anger and grief, awareness and compassion: they go out to make plans with people who knew Herod how best to kill Jesus. His choice is compassion. Theirs is a violence plotted with bitter enemies in their fight for the heart and soul of their people.

Does this make you sad? It makes me sad. Not depressed, just sad. When I look upon or paint an image of Christ on the cross, I know as I have known since the Sisters of Mercy did their thing for me at St. Ann School, that he died for **my** sins.

In my one summer as a hospital chaplain, I got to know a delightful man who grew up as a Jew in a Catholic neighborhood. The kids beat him up, stole his lunch, and said ugly things to him about Jews. He had become convinced that we named as *Judas* the one who betrayed Jesus because *Judas* sounds like *Jew*.

I apologized to him, but he did not want my apologies. He was given pause when I told him that whenever I heard the name Judas, what entered my mind was that *Judas* represents me, because Jesus died for my sins. It had never occurred to me how a Jewish kid in a Catholic neighborhood might hear the name *Judas* in a different way. As I write this, I am feeling the bond of compassion that I felt that day with him.

What can I do when I am angry with even my brother? This is not theoretical for me. Some years ago God graced me with a way to pray this. With the gift of imagination, I stand next to the brother, with him in front of our God, and I say something like:

Loving Abba, this is my brother,
*   and you know my feelings and our entire story.*
Lord, I believe that as you created me in your image,
*   so too you created my brother in your image.*
Lord, created in your image? Hard time seeing it!
*   But you alone see everything in both of our hearts.*
Lord, I don't want to see everything you see,
*   because I am not yet ready for it all,*
*   but could you show me something today of how*
*   my brother and I are both created in your image?*
*   Help me to feel my anger with grief and compassion,*
*   knowing as did your Son whom they wanted to kill,*
*   that we are all broken, wounded in our humanity.*

Another religious practice, if I may be a pharisee, is to offer intercessory prayer for myself and the person with whom I am angry. Gifts that make this possible are:
(1) faith in God's love for all people,
(2) the truth that it is not possible for me to know everything going on in the heart of another person,
(3) the liklihood that God alone knows what is blocking the person with whom I am angry from being open to reconciliation or health, and (gulp)
(4) even the grace of accepting that the real problem may be me and not the other.

Anger is righteous only when I am in the right. Truly, how often am I completely just and righteous? Don't answer that. Almost always I am responsible at least partially for what has gone wrong whether by trying to control a person or a situation or by having unrealistic expectations of myself.* Even a truly innocent victim will eventually need the healing of the emotion of anger that comes only in forgiving.

If I am graced with the gift of awareness that the one with whom I am angry is, like me, created in God's own image, adopted as God's own daughter or son, then I might be ready for intercessory prayer. I think of intercessory prayer as a way to give to God permission to do what God wants to do.

I am not talking out of both sides of my mouth. If I am in an unhealthy place in my life, I might not be free or capable of asking God for the help I need, and which I desire without even knowing it. I might be so angry with God as to ask God to just leave me alone. God respects my freedom. However, if my friend, or my enemy, asks God to intercede, to make the healing touch that God already wants to make, then God can respect the freedom of my friend or of my enemy, and then freely heal me.

* (Remember, in any kind of child abuse, the adult is **always** the one responsible.)

The Church teaches with wisdom that each passage of sacred scripture is best read in the the context of **all** of scripture. As you think of our story of the anger-grief of Jesus, what other passages of the Bible or words from our faith tradition come to mind? Here are some to which I am drawn:

You have heard that it was said to your ancestors, *'You shall not kill..."* *But I say to you,* don't stay angry with your brother or call him *raqa* (an imbecile or a blockhead) (Mt 5:21-22). The theologian and author of Ephesians adds: *Be angry but do not sin; do not let the sun set on your anger* (Ephesians 4:26). I find as helpful supports to this teaching two images from the Wisdom Book of Sirach: *Wrath and anger are hateful things, yet the sinner hugs them tight* (Sirach 27:30), and *If you blow upon a spark, it quickens into flame, if you spit on it, it dies out; yet both you do with your mouth* (Sirach 28:12). In Jesus' turning there is time. The time it takes for him to turn is time enough for his anger to be overcome with healing grief. So often, my choice is to feed the anger with words of fertilizer, water and sun (to mix metaphors), to do whatever it takes to keep the spark of anger alive, even to the point of pleasure. Jesus shows us a different way.

Go first and be reconciled with your brother, and then come and offer your gift at the altar (Mt 5:24). Jesus calls us to make peace. Few of us want this job. We have it anyway.

You have heard that it was said, 'You shall love your neighbor and hate your enemy (see Leviticus 19:18), *but I say to you, love your enemies, and pray for those who persecute you, that you may be children of your heavenly Father, for he makes his sun rise on the bad and the good, and causes rain to fall on the just and the unjust* (Mt 5:43-45). An old friend still says this is the most difficult of all of the teachings of Jesus. I cannot do it on my own. I cannot do it without God's grace. I can ask God for that grace.

Words of scripture we know as the Lord's Prayer say so much of what Jesus has taught us:
...And forgive us...as we forgive... (Mt 6:12).
How much of our lives do we spend trying to find another way? This is the way.

St. Paul's excellent teaching is also a huge help:
If your enemy is hungry, feed him (Romans 12:20). Paul's practical advice is as effective as it is difficult.

And the theologian Pope John Paul II, after the September 11, 2001 attack, said to the world: *No peace without justice... no justice without forgiveness...,* building on Pope Paul VI's often quoted maxim: *If you want peace, work for justice.* Adding *forgiveness* to Paul VI's maxim, John Paul II speaks an essential truth. One of my teachers in the Holy Land was a priest who had spent the bulk of his adult life as a counselor to teenagers, but who was then a peace worker for the United Nations. He used to say that there would not be peace in the Middle East until somebody with courage willingly ended the cycle of retaliation by forgiving. It hit me one day, listening to him, how central is forgiveness to the Christian identity.

At the sacrament of Baptism, the one made newly wet *in the name of the Father and of the Son and of the Holy Spirit* (Mt 28:19) is "anointed" (which is what the word *Christ* means) with oil, and then given this message of our vocation:

> *As Jesus Christ was anointed priest, prophet and king,*
> *so may you live always as a member of his body...*

As a **prophet**, the Christian will be called to proclaim a truth to somebody who God wants to hear that truth, and to speak that truth with compassion. As a **king or queen**, the Christian will be called to use his or her gifts, abilities, strengths and charisms in service of humanity, sometimes as leader, always as a servant. As a **priest**, the Christian will be called to pray and forgive. We cannot wriggle out of our vocation of forgiveness. When the apostles were bluntly told of their vocation to forgive, not seven or seventy times, but seven times seventy times, their response was from the gut: *Increase our faith!* (Luke 17:5).

We too ask our Lord and Savior (who entered human history as Son of God and Son of Man to dwell in our midst, share our experience, and show us the way; who gave himself completely in his teaching and preaching and healing ministry even to dying for us on the cross; who was raised from the dead, appeared to the women and the apostles and the disciples who recognized him in the breaking of the bread (Lk 24:31); who having told Mary Magdalene to not cling to him, ascended to the Father and with the Father sent their Holy Spirit upon the Church beginning at Pentecost and continuing even to this very day) we too can ask for the grace we know we will need to forgive and to keep on forgiving, by echoing the apostles:

Lord, increase our faith!

God wants us to participate in this. Here is one
more key-to-the-lock forgiveness story:

Toward the end of the gospel of John, the church
is gathered in fear, in the upper room, behind doors
locked tight. Afraid. Jesus breaks through their fear
and the locked doors, and convinces them he is alive.
(Was Mary offering intercessory prayer for them?)
He then does something quite remarkable:

Jesus **breathes** on them, saying,

Receive the holy Spirit.
Whose sins you forgive are forgiven them, and
whose sins you retain are retained" (John 20:22b,23).

There is a context to the Upper Room story: we call
it Good Friday. On the cross, Jesus would have been
pulling himself up through the pain to take another
breath. The offical cause of death of most people who
were crucified was suffocation, when they no longer
had the strength to pull themselves up to breathe.
In the second Genesis story of creation, God breathed
the breath of life into Adam. We suffocated the Son,
who then breathes the Holy Spirit on us.

This Easter story is one of the sources of our
sacrament of reconciliation, indeed. It speaks also
a truth for all people, one by one. We are free. We
may choose to hold onto the unforgiven, but to do so
is to stay enslaved. We have been given by God the
freedom, and by the Son the power, and by their
Spirit the grace, to forgive. Embrace your humanity;
hear the divinity of Christ within you; breathe in the
Holy Spirit who has come to you. Accept the healing
that will let you throw out coping. Breathe. Breathe
deeply the freedom and power given you by our God.

☦

☩

In the name of the Father
and of the Son
and of the Holy Breath of God.
Lord Jesus, Son of God and son of Mary,
pattern of my life,
promise and image of who I am called to be,
help me to know and hold my anger
with grief that may turn it to compassion.
Risen Lord, with our Father,
keep breathing your Holy Spirit
over and into me
and to all who would be enemies
the desire and the power
to forgive.
Thanks be to you,
God of the universe.

☩

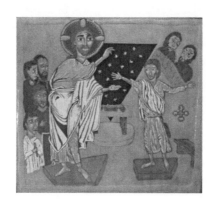

...looking   *and grieved*
around   *at their*
at them   *hardness*
with anger   *of heart...*

These reflections are a remembrance of many short conversations with people of faith, most often in the sacrament of reconciliation. Since you have read this far perhaps you are ready for some of whatever healing with which the one God, Father, Son and Spirit, wishes to touch you. I invite you to find a quiet place, sit, breathe, and simply ask for the Lord's healing touch. I will be praying for your healing and for all blessings.

- Fr. Steve Wolf

Acknowledgments

Page 21: St. Ignatius of Loyola, *The Spiritual Exercises,*
especially paragraphs 122-125. The best way to
experience the exercises is on an individually directed
retreat. Find Jesuit retreat centers at www.jesuit.org.

Page 23: *Monty Python's Life of Brian,* 1979, 94 minutes,
Brian is born on the original Christmas, in the stable
next door. Rated R, not for children, No Way, much
of the bad language is terribly unnecessary. The humor
is masterful. My report is from weak memory; in the
movie the man was a leper instead of a cripple:

Ex-Leper: Okay, sir, my final offer: half a shekel for an old
ex-leper?

Brian: Did you say "ex-leper"?

Ex-Leper: That's right, sir, 16 years behind a veil and proud of it.

Brian: Well, what happened?

Ex-Leper: Oh, cured, sir.

Brian: Cured?

Ex-Leper: Yes sir, bloody miracle, sir. Bless you!

Brian: Who cured you?

Ex-Leper: Jesus did, sir. I was hopping along, minding my
own business, all of a sudden, up he comes, cures me!
One minute I'm a leper with a trade, next minute my
livelihood's gone. Not so much as a by-your-leave!
"You're cured, mate." Bloody do-gooder.

Brian: Well, why don't you go and tell him you want to be a
leper again?

Ex-Leper: Uh, I could do that sir, yeah. Yeah, I could do that
I suppose. What I was thinking was I was going to ask
him if he could make me a bit lame in one leg during the
middle of the week. You know, something beggable,
but not leprosy, which is a pain in the...

Brian: There you are.

Ex-Leper: Half a dinare for me bloody life story?

Brian: There's no pleasing some people.

Ex-Leper: That's just what Jesus said, sir.

Page 24: *citadel of psychic safety,* Ted Peters, *Sin: Radical
Evil in Soul & Society,* 1999.

Page 24: *self-complacent finitude,* Paul Tillich, *The Religious
Situation,* 1925.

Page 29: Steve Wolf, *Letter of the Pharisee,* from a
homework assignment at Mundelein Seminary.

Page 34: *anger, grief,* from *Webster's New World Dictionary.* Friend and scholar, James Pratt, S.J. is the first who told me that the phrase can also mean that *his bowels turned inward,* a way to also understand *compassion.*

Page 35: *God on his poppa's side...,* Eugene LaVerdierre. Bill Huebsch puts it this way in *A Spirituality of Wholeness,* Twenty-Third Publications, 1988:

> We are not alone. And Jesus was not alone either. We often misunderstand this in the gospels. We think, Well, Jesus was God. He was all powerful. He didn't have to deal with life the way I do...
>
> Jesus is God. No doubt about it. But he is also human, very human, completely human, humanly human.
>
> He ate, drank, slept, urinated, sweated, wept, worried, sang, told stories, was aroused, worked, got blisters, made mistakes, and generally was a regular type of guy.
>
> Jesus was human and he faced all that humans face. He wasn't half human and half divine, Gene LaVerdiere has pointed out, you know, sort of human on his mother's side and divine on his father's side!
>
> No. He was fully human and fully divine.
> This is mysterious and hard to understand, but it is also very important.

Page 36: *hardness,* from *Strong's Concordance*

Page 38: One example of this is in Thomas Merton, *Learning To Love, Journals, Volume 6,* Christine M. Bochen, Editor, San Francisco: HarperSanFrancisco, 1998, pg. 320:

One...work(s) at solitude, not by putting fences around oneself, but by destroying all fences and throwing away all the disguises, getting down to the naked core of one's inmost desire, which is the desire of liberty-reality...to be real in the freedom which reality gives when one is rightly related to it.

Page 43: *no peace without justice; no justice without forgiveness,* Pope John Paul II, *Message for the Celebration of the World Day of Peace,* January 1, 2002.

If you want peace, work for justice, Pope Paul VI, *Message for the Celebration of the Day of Peace,* January 1, 1972, also attributed to H. L. Mencken, 1880-1956, perhaps a wise antidote to the Latin maxim, *if you want peace, prepare for war.*

Page 44: *as Christ was anointed...,* ICEL, *Rite of Baptism for Children,* paragraph 125.

A Reader's Question

A reader has asked if I have more to say about grief.

OK, you are correct. This book has really been about anger, and less about grief. I often call myself a very slow griever. Not a problem; we all do it differently. Unique grieving is wrapped up in the unique way each of us is made in God's image. If the 5 steps of grief are on target (denial, anger, bargaining, depression, and acceptance), anger is for me the hardest part. So let's be easy on each other with how we grieve, and put this too in the strong hands of the Lord.

My favorite saying about grief touches the core of healing to be found in forgiveness. It is from a graphic tale of a man who was abused as a teen, who discovered what I know as sanity in a friend's response, "that's tricky" to his all-of-a-sudden declaration: "It's letting go of the sense that the past should have been any different or better" (Martin Moran, *The Tricky Part,* Vintage Books/AnchorBooks, 2005). Mr. Moran's inspiration is the best I know to offer, except for the word of God to which I tether my soul on days of depression. These words too I offer:

SCRIPTURE IN HEALTH AND IN HEALING

	MORNINGS	EVENINGS
Sunday	Psalm 100, Mark 16:5-6	Psalm 23; 1 Corinthians 15:3-8
Monday	Ps 42:1-6a; Matthew 8:1-3	Psalm 121; Ezekiel 36:24-28
Tuesday	Ps 139:1-10; Mark 3:1-5	Psalm 84:1-9; Ephesians 2:19-22
Wednesday	Ps 63:1-8; Romans 8:22-27	Psalm 131; Philippians 2:5-11
Thursday	Ps 86:1-7,11; Rom 8:14-17	Psalm 126; Luke 6:17-19
Friday	Ps 51:10-19; Luke 17:20-21	Psalm 65:4,9-13; John 14:1-7
Saturday	Psalm 46; Ephesians 3:16-22	Psalm 147:1-11; Matt 8:23-27

The Story, One More Time

1   *Again Jesus entered the synagogue.*
There was a man there
who had a withered hand.

2   *They watched him closely*
to see if he would cure him on the sabbath
so that they might accuse him.

3   *He said to the man with the withered hand,*
"Come up here before us."

4   *Then he said to them,*
"Is it lawful to do good on the sabbath
rather than to do evil,
to save life rather than destroy it?"
But they remained silent.

5   *Looking around at them with anger*
and grieved at their hardness of heart,
he said to the man,
"Stretch out your hand."
He stretched it out and his hand was restored.

6   *The Pharisees went out*
and immediately took counsel with the Herodians
against him to put him to death.

Mark 3:1-6

Thanks be to Deacon Fred Bourland and his FIAT group for the Ponder Page questions on pages 59 and 61.

1. How have I seen religious rules or institutions hurt people? What causes that?

2. Have I ever felt angry at a church or religious institution? Why? How has that experience affected me?

3. Did I grow up with any Sunday restrictions? Do I still honor them?

4. Which of my parents' rules did I break most often?

5. Have I ever experienced conflict on how to spend my "Sabbath" day?

6. What made Jesus so upset with the Pharisees in the synagogue?

7. What made the Pharisees so upset with Jesus?

8. What does "Sabbath" mean to me?

21 *You have heard*
that it was said to your ancestors,
  'You shall not kill;
   and whoever kills will be liable to judgment.'
22 *But I say to you,*
whoever is angry with his brother
will be liable to judgment,
and whoever says to his brother, 'Raqa,'
will be answerable to the Sanhedrin,
and whoever says, 'You fool,"
will be liable to fiery Gehenna…"

Matthew 5:21-22

13,14 *…Jesus went up to Jerusalem. He found in the*
temple area those who sold oxen, sheep, and doves,
as well as the money-changers seated there.
15 *He made a whip out of cords and drove them all*
out of the temple area, with the sheep and oxen,
and spilled the coins of the money-changers and
16 *overturned their tables, and to those who sold doves*
he said, "Take these out of here,
and stop making my Father's house a marketplace."
17 *His disciples recalled the words of scripture,*
*" **Zeal** for your house will consume me."*

John 2:13b-17 (*Zeal* is from Psalm 69:10)

60

1. What is the best advice I have been given for dealing with anger?

2. Since all of us experience anger, what is Jesus saying to us here?

3. Have I ever gotten angry with God when someone I love goes through hard times?

4. Is it a sin to be angry with God?

5. What do I do when I am angry with God?

1. How might the once useful practice of selling sacrificial animals have deteriorated into a racket? Why else was Jesus probably angry?

2. As one of the sellers, how would I feel about what Jesus did in the temple area?

3. As one of the disciples, how would I feel?

4. If I compare my spiritual life to the rooms of a house, which room might Jesus want to clean up?

Thanks That Be

It takes the help of many souls for a parish priest to goof off for five whole months. I am grateful for the sabbatical, but especially for the gift of these good people:

- The parishioners of St. Stephen Catholic Community in Hermitage, Old Hickory and Mt. Juliet, Tennessee
- Parish staff: Barb Couturier, Cecilia Thomas, Youth Minister Angie Bosio, Ministries Coordinator Francie Duffield, RCIA Director Mary Craven, DRE Greg Karn, Music Director Scott Goudeau, Children Initiation Director Connie Blevins, Life Teen Band Leader Renee Campbell, Nursery Director Jaime Boyer, and Facilities Maintenance Staff Debby White, Allen Shankle, Gary Anderson, and Romey Baltz
- Rev. Theophilus Ebulueme, Head Sacristan Luis Bustillos, and Ed English
- Deacons Fred Bourland, Mickey Rose, Hans Toecker, and Jim Batcheldor
- Most Rev. David R. Choby, Bishop of Nashville and Sister Kathleen Flood, O.P.
- 2008 Parish Council Co-chairs John Castner & Craig Lewis; Youth Reps: Alec Ozminski & Ian Reding, Worship: Jim Simpson, Teresa Lundberg, & Cassie Kinsman; Word: John Reding, Erin Muldoon, & Danny Ford; Service: Gary Rabideau, Nicki Ballard & Jillian Hinesley; Vocation: Dennis Kaney, Katie Humphrey, & Catherine Black; Evangelization: Kathy Sullivan, Linda Norfleet, & Wil Heidorn; Stewardship: Kathy Walsh, Jim Mattingly, & Carly McMahon; Secretary: Rickie McQueen
- Priests of the Community of Passionists who assisted at Sunday Masses and Rev. Donald Webber, CP, Provincial, who gave his permission
- Ken Schmitt, daughter Annie, and the Passionist Partners of Nashville
- Tom Samoray, Director of Vocation Awareness and Young Adult Ministry
- All the Trappist monks of the Monastery of the Holy Spirit in Conyers, Georgia, including Brother Michael, Fr. James Stephen, Fr. Tom Francis, Fr. Anthony, Fr. Gerard, Abbot Francis Michael, OCSO, and the outstanding guest house staff
- The Mercy Center in Colorado Springs, CO, especially Josie Gallegos, Donna DeBartolo, Bill Winaski, Margaret Henson, and Heidi Miller
- The Institute for Continuing Theological Education (ICTE) of the North American College in Rome, especially Rev. Michael Wensing in his first semester as director, great teachers including Rev. Craig Morrison, O.Carm., Msgr. James Moroney, Rev. Daniel Mueggenborg, Rev. Mark Attard, O.Carm., and what a bunch of brother priests: Joe Badding, Gerry Bechard, Jim Byers, John Capuci, Jim Carlson, Michael De Verteuil, Craig Eilerman, Don Greenhalgh, Steve Hornat, SSE, John Keefe, Joe Kelly, Bernard Kiely, Robert Lariviere, James Le, Larry McBride, Jim McClintock, Gary Meier, Michael Motta, Daniel Nascimento, Moses Ou'ou, Jay Peterson, Francis Van Pham Phuong, Gerard Pilon, James Singler, Andrzej Skizypiec, Pius To'omae and Richard Wise, tour guide extraordinaire Dr. Elizabeth Lev, and Carol Salfa
- friends and fellow travellers on the journey: James Dylan Myers, Mike Dunne and the baseball trip gang, Rev. Brian Schieber, fellow Merton freak Ken Voiles, Deacon Rob and Maria Montini, Art Guys Michael Galbreth and Jack Massing, Rainey and Tennessee Samuel Galbreth, Rev. James F.X. Pratt, SJ, and Rev. Bill Vollmer
- and you too, Lord: Thank You!

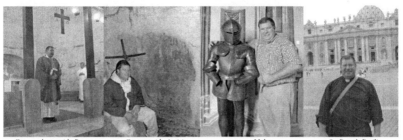

Catacombs outside Rome   Cave outside Assisi   Malta   St. Peter's Basilic

Stephen Joseph Wolf is a parish priest in the Diocese of Nashville, where he grew up a West Nashville street urchin, the second of eight sons of Charlie and Jeanette. Schooled at St. Ann, Father Ryan High School, Middle Tennessee State University *MTSU,* with an MBA from Belmont University, and as a Certified Public Accountant with Carter, Young, Wolf & Dahlhauser, P.C, after 14 tax seasons, then 5 years at Mundelein Seminary in Chicago, and ordained in 1997, he has served as Master of Ceremonies, Director of Vocation Formation, on the Presbyteral Council, and on the Nashville Boards of Catholic Charities and NCCJ. He is pastor and spiritual director at St. Stephen Catholic Community in Hermitage, Old Hickory and Mt. Juliet, and active in Congregations Offering a Living Wage *COLW* and the Tennessee Coalition to Abolish State Killing *TCASK.* **Anger-Grief the Jesus Way** was written while on sabbatical at the Monastery of the Holy Spirit in Conyers, Georgia, at the Mercy Center in Colorado Springs, and at North American College in Rome, with gratitude. Other works include *Money and Freedom: the New American Game* (1992) with Eric Dahlhauser, CPA, *The Passion Narratives* (2006), *Psalm Songs* (2003-2008), and *God's Money* (2008). Prayer books include *In Health and In Healing, Hinge Hours Experiment* (4 vol.), and *Resurrection Trail.*

Printed in the United States
152174LV00002B/1/P